Occupational Therapy:
Ten Simple Steps to Independent Contracting

Tomeico Faison, CEO, OTR/L

Business Consultant and Certified Business Coach

Ten Simple Steps to Independent Contracting

About Tomeico- Tomeico Faison is an occupational therapist and an entrepreneurial guru. She has helped over 50 health and human service professionals start and grow businesses. She has grown her business from scratch to a company grossing more than half a million dollars in sales annually with a focus on niche underserved populations, such as persons with mental illness, developmental disabilities and low vision. She believes in the power of purpose and service and is dedicated to being a leading educator and advocate for health and human service entrepreneurs. Contact Tomeico Faison today for a FREE 30 minute initial consultative or coaching session!

Visit www.faisonconsulting.com for more information.

Why I wrote this booklet:

I have been an occupational therapist since 2001 and have been contracting since 2003. Since I have been contracting, I have had numerous therapists ask me specific questions about becoming contractors or owning their own businesses. Many of these therapists believe that contracting is a very difficult thing to do and are amazed that I started contracting shortly after becoming a therapist. I am often drilled with questions regarding how one gets started as an independent contractor. Most of the time I am able to talk to them about the process but not always. Time is precious and I am truly a busy lady. However, I believe in helping others and have found the remedy to sharing my basic knowledge about becoming an independent contractor in an efficient manner. The remedy is this information booklet, workshops and consultation and coaching services. This booklet consists of the basic steps to becoming an independent contractor for therapists. If you are looking for a booklet about opening up your own outpatient therapy practice or home health agency, then this is not the booklet for you. This booklet focuses on the business of independent contracting and is based on my personal success with this type of practice. I am sharing with my audience a simple way to be self-employed as a contractor with other businesses, such as the outpatient therapy practices or home health agencies. Independent contracting has certainly been a blessing for me and I hope that my knowledge can help you.

Therapeutic Solutions has now expanded well beyond solely providing contractual services and has added more niche market services, such as in-home low vision services, group home consultation, community mental health services, geriatric social work services, etc. Additionally, I recently created a nonprofit to assist persons who need services but have limited financial resources. Although, we have expanded and we understand many therapists have a desire to go into specialized niche markets, independent contracting has proven to be the simplest form of self-employment and is an excellent start for therapists who are interested in testing the waters of the world of entrepreneurship!

Disclaimer

The information in this booklet is based on the personal perspectives and experiences of the author, Tomeico Faison and are for educational purposes only. The author is a business consultant and coach for health and human services professionals interested in independent contracting and does not provide legal and financial advice. The information is for educational purposes only and is not intended to replace the advice from credentialed professionals, such as attorneys and accountants. The information is also not intended to replace the contract agency's requirements.

No parts of this booklet can be copied without the written permission of Tomeico Faison.

Ten Simple Steps to Independent Contracting

Table of Contents

Why I wrote this booklet: ii

Disclaimer   iv

Steps   1

Step 1-Find Out if You Really Want to be an Independent Contractor   2

Step 2-Follow Your Passion...Where There is A Need, Passions Bring Pleasure   8

STEP # 3- Decide To Be Incorporated or Not To Be Incorporated   12

Step 4-Get Insured!   20

Step 5: An Accountant and Attorney are Your Friends-Develop a Rapport   24

Step 6-Determine Your Rate-What's the Plan?   27

Step 7: Review or Write Your Contracts   31

Step 8-Marketing   32

STEP 9-Consider Hiring Subcontractors if You Want to Expand   35

Step 10-Go Get Some Contacts!!!   38

Final Thoughts: 42

Steps

Step 1-Find Out if You Really Want to Be an Independent Contractor Step 2-Follow Your Passion...Where There is a Need.

Step 3-Decide to Be Incorporated or Not to be Incorporated Step 4-Get Insured.

Step 5-An Accountant and Attorney are Your Friends Step 6-Determine Your Rate and What's the Plan?

Step 7-Review or Write Your Contracts Step 8-Marketing-Low Cost Options.

Step 9-Consider Hiring Subcontractors if You Want to Expand Step 10-Go Get Some Contracts.

Step 1-Find Out if You Really Want to be an Independent Contractor

Independent Contractor Definition

In order to become an independent contractor, one obviously needs to know the definition of an independent contractor. Note the following definitions below.

"INDEPENDENT CONTRACTOR- A person or business who performs services for another person under an express or implied agreement and who is not subject to the other's control, or right to control, the manner and means of performing the services; not as an employee. One who engages an independent contractor is not liable to others for the acts or omissions of the independent contractor."

http://www.lectlaw.com/def/i028.htm

*General rule-the individual is an independent contractor if the person for whom the services are performed has control over the result of the work, not the method of accomplishing the results.

http://www.irs.gov/

In other words, as an independent contractor your method of accomplishing results may not be dictated by the contracting agency. For example, I contract with a chain of local group homes. My job is to provide occupational therapy services as needed but there is no one to tell me how I am supposed to write my progress notes or conduct my evaluations. I am independent in terms of how the services are provided. The agency is only interested in the result—provision of competent services that meet the consumers' needs. However, some agencies have specific policies and procedures and compliance is required. Control over method of service provision will vary depending upon settings and can range from no control or direction to required compliance with rigid policies and procedures.

Employee versus Contractor

One question that is commonly asked of me is, "What is the difference between an independent contractor and an employee?" Some of the basic differences I have noted are in the table below.

Employee	Independent Contractor (IC)
Therapist is working for an agency or company	Therapist is self-employed and providing services for a company or agency
Employer deducts taxes from earnings	IC is responsible for paying all taxes to the appropriate government agencies
Employer provides liability coverage	IC is responsible for liability coverage

Ten Simple Steps to Independent Contracting

Employer provides workers compensation coverage	IC is responsible for worker's compensation coverage which may or may not be required by contracting agency and/or state
Salary is typically predetermined by employer	Salary is typically negotiated between IC and contract agency
Schedule is typically predetermined by employer	Schedule is typically negotiated between IC and contract agency
Duties are defined in a drop description	Duties are defined in a contract agreement
Job is typically indefinite unless otherwise specified	Job is typically time limited as specified in the contract agreement. Contract agency typically reserves the right to terminate the contract at anytime for any reason providing a minimum of a 30-day notice. IC also has the right to terminate the contract at anytime for any reason providing a minimum of a 30-day notice.
Pay schedule is typically consistent	Pay schedule may vary as long as the IC is paid within a provided time frame as specified in the contract agreement Ex. "IC will be paid within 30 days of receipt of invoice."

See irs.gov for more information about employees versus independent contractors. Reference: irs.gov

PRN versus Contract

Another question that I am typically asked is, "What is the difference between a pro rate nada (PRN) employee and a contract worker. As a PRN worker you are an employee. Thus, your employer is responsible for deducting taxes and providing liability insurance coverage. In contrast, taxes and liability insurance are a contractor's personal responsibility. Another big difference between PRN and contract work is that PRN employees work "as needed" and contract workers work according to the hours deemed necessary in the contract agreement. As a PRN employee, you may work 20 hours one week and no hours at all for the next two weeks, dependent upon the need. However, as a contract worker, you will likely have a certain minimum amount of consistent weekly hours as stated in your contract agreement. Additionally, as a PRN employee you always have the option to reject hours when offered. As an independent contractor, you have agreed to work the provided hours stated in the contract and are bound to the contract terms.

Entrepreneurship Assessment

Now that you know the definition of an IC and some of the differences between an IC and an employee, you should think about your ability to handle entrepreneurship. I was born to be a small business owner. I love entrepreneurship so much that I literally think of new businesses daily. My mind operates like a business owner and not an employee. In fact, I am now doing business consultation because I cannot possibly start-up every business that comes to my mind—although I have tried at times. My goal now however is to help inspire others to start up some of these innovative businesses so that I can see more dreams turn into realities and more needs being met in our communities. Once I decided to write and provide consultative business services, I immediately dropped some of my direct contract work. When work is dropped, I am always presented with risk of not replacing the lost income. However, I am a risk taker and this personality characteristic helps me to be flexible and dealwith unpredictable situations. Several therapists have told me that they do not understand how I can work as a contractor when there is always the possibility of not having work. Some of these therapists have shared that their personality is a better fit for consistent stable employment. Although I am always encouraging entrepreneurship, I respect persons who understand their limitations and know that entrepreneurship may bring more stress to their lives than excitement. As an IC you are self-employed and thus, you will need to examine your personality characteristics to help you decide if contracting is right for you. You may also want to consider partnering with someone who may be more of risk taker. With partners, one's weaknesses can be another person's strengths.

Entrepreneurship Assessment

Ask yourself the following questions to help you decide if contracting is for you.

1. Are you a risk taker?
2. Are you flexible? Are you willing to commute? Are you willing to work in different practice settings?
3. Does your financial situation allow you to have times of lack of employment or late payments? Can you handle getting paid late occasionally?
4. Do you like to network? Are you a person who enjoys meeting new people?

5. Are you organized? Can you make your own schedule and accomplish the required job duties without direct supervision?
6. Are you a good financial manager? Can you stay within the required contract budget?
7. Can you keep good records? Can you keep files of incoming and outgoing expenses and invoice sheets?
8. Can you work independently? Can you work without other therapists being around and without supervision?
9. Are you ambitious? Do you work hard? Are you innovative?
10. Are you good at what you do? Do you have a good reputation as a therapist? Do you have good references?

Entrepreneurship Assessment

Answering ten questions obviously is not the sole assessment that one needs to take to determine if he/she should become an entrepreneur. Understanding your purpose and the best means to accomplish this purpose is the best way to determine if you need to be an entrepreneur. However, examining the answers to these questions is part of a good start to this assessment process. If you answered "no" more than you answered "yes", you may want to consider other options, partnering with others or getting consultation and coaching services to help you overcome challenges. However, if you answered "yes" to more questions than you answered "no", you may already be seasoned to become an entrepreneur but will still need to address the challenges noted through entrepreneurial support resources, such as workshops, coaching and consultation.

Step 2-Follow Your Passion...Where There is A Need, Passions Bring Pleasure

This second step is critical in regards to maintaining motivation while working as an independent contractor. If you follow your passion, you are less likely to become unmotivated because you will enjoy what you are doing. At one point, I took almost every contract opportunity that came my way. I was working at skilled nursing facilities, a psychiatric institution and at group homes. I quickly found myself working mostly at the psychiatric institution and at the group homes with clients who were considered "high functioning" with mild mental impairments. My passion is in mental health and geriatrics. I found that I was not very motivated to work with persons with severe physical impairments. Whenever I got a phone call from a group home supervisor regarding splints or range of motion, it took a lot of energy to respond. On the other hand, whenever I got a call from a group home supervisor regarding helping a consumer learn to manage a budget, I was elated and eager to respond to the referral.

When I realized that my passion was truly for the geriatric population and persons with mental health diagnoses, I began to discontinue contracts that did not allow me to follow my passions or select subcontractors who were interested in those practice areas. Think about the population and setting that you would like to work most. Then come up with a list (1-6) which includes most passionate to least passionate work settings. Consider aspects of the setting that would cause you to be more or less passionate about your work. For example, I love working in a person's natural setting, such as with home health. However, I hate traffic and extensive day-to-day travel. I am always getting lost— even with a navigation system in my car! Weigh the pros and cons of the settings you enjoy and come up with a list of contract work options.

Passion Brings Pleasure Sometimes....

If you focus on what you love and were made to do, when things get hard you will persevere. Passion brings pleasure only sometimes. Other times, you may be frustrated with politics, financial management, contract negotiation and other factors that turn black hairs grey. However, your passionate commitment to your purpose will help you presson.

Your Top Six List:

1.

2.

3.

4.

5.

6.

I Dream of a Business...........

What does your dream independent contracting work look like? Write, Draw, Dream....

There Must Be a Need in Order to Succeed

Lastly but certainly not least, you will need to determine if there is a need for independent contracting in the areas in which you are willing to work. It makes no sense to decide to become an IC and go after a passion if there are no employers who have a need or desire for contract services. You will need to scan your potential work environment and do a mini-needs assessment. Here are some examples of things I looked at before becoming an IC.

- Sample of Occupational Therapy Job Market Assessment
    - Checked the Occupational Outlook Handbook
    - Scanned the local newspaper weekly
    - Looked at job opening in Advance magazine
    - Looked at job openings on the NC Occupational Therapy Website and American Occupational Therapy Association Website
    - Contacted local employers and asked supervisors if they would be willing to hire a contractor for services
    - Mailed out brochures to group home agencies
    - Researched health trends, such as increase aging population, increase in community-based services for children, growing MR/DD population etc.

- Spoke with other independent contractors in rehabilitation fields(other occupational therapists, speech therapists, physical therapists)

Other Things to Do:

- Check out the competition-Who else is doing what you want to do?
- Research the competition and look for service gaps
- Look at health care trends (example: state mental health reform, increase population)
- Collaborate with the Small Business Administration (SBA) and the local Chamber of Commerce, the Federal Government, SCORE and local community colleges

STEP # 3- Decide To Be Incorporated or Not To Be Incorporated

As an IC, you can work under your personal name and social security or incorporate a business and work under the business name and the business's employment identification number (EIN).

If You Decide Not to Be Incorporated Sole Proprietorship "A sole proprietor is someone who owns an unincorporated business himself or herself." (www.irs.gov)

Some people choose not to be incorporated because they dislike the extra paperwork requirements and regulations. Sole proprietorship is the simplest type of business in existence. There are less start-up costs, documentation requirements and regulations if you are not incorporated. However, you are personally liable for your work and thus, your personal assets are at risk. Since you and the business are one in the same then you can be sued for any of your personal possessions (house, cars, etc.) Additionally, if you are married your spouses' assets may also be at risk. If you however prefer to be a sole proprietor due to the simplicity that it affords, you will follow the steps below.

- You can use your LEGAL name without filing any paperwork
- If you choose to use another name, you will need to contact your county's Register of Deeds for specifics. Go to your state secretary of state's page and search Register of Deeds
- You will fill out a W-9 form for tax purposes if you are working for other companies

Business Structures

- Taxes will not be withheld from your paycheck. Taxes will be your responsibility.
- You will be responsible for keeping up with your income and expenses
- You will use your name and social security number on the W-9form
- You will need to check with your county and city zoning agencies to determine if you need any special permits, such as a home office permit if you will be using a home office
- You will be considered a 1099 worker if you are contracting with an agency meaning that at the end of the year, you will receive a 1099 form stating your total income earned versus a W-2 (which is as you know the tax form you receive as an employee at the end of the year)

"Partnership-A partnership is a relationship existing between two or more people who join to carry on a trade or business. Each person contributes money, property, labor or skill and expects to share in the profits and losses of the business." (www.irs.gov).

Written agreements regarding the relationship are recommended. Partnerships don't pay taxes but instead file a return that is informational. Individual partners report their personal share of profits and losses on their personal return (www.sba.gov).

What is a Corporation?

"A corporation is a separate legal entity that exists independently from its owners. A corporation is created and comes into existence when articles of incorporation (charter or certificate of incorporation in certain states) are filed with the proscribed fees, and accepted by the proper state authority."

http://www.incorporation-e.com/item-1.htm

Business Structures

If You Decide to Become Incorporated

You might ask, "Why might you become incorporated in the first place? "Becoming incorporated gives you certain tax advantages depending on the type of corporation you choose. However, the main reason I chose to become incorporated is because I wanted to keep my personal assets separate from my business assets. My company is a limited liability corporation (LLC) and therefore my business is liable for my work, not me personally and thus, my personal assets are protected more. In other words, if my business is sued then I would be sued for business assets and my personal assets are at less risk.

Below are a few brief descriptions of some basic corporation structures from the sba.gov website. I recommend taking a look at the www.sba.gov website to learn more about types of corporations, including their perspective on pros and cons. If you want more specific information, you may also want to sit down with an attorney and accountant (many do free initial consultations) who can go over legalities and tax information respectively, based on corporation status.

Basic Structures

Limited Liability Company (LLC)

"The LLC is generally considered advantageous for small businesses because it combines the limited personal liability feature of a corporation with the tax advantages of a partnership and sole proprietorship. Profits and losses can be passed through the company to its members or the LLC can elect to be taxed like a corporation. LLCs do not have stock and are not required to observe corporate formalities. Owners are called members, and the LLC is managed by these members or by appointed managers."

(www.sba.gov)

C Corporation (Inc. or Ltd.)

"This is a complex business structure with more startup costs than many other forms. A corporation is a legal entity separate from its owners, who own shares of stock in the company. Corporations can be created for profit or nonprofit purposes and may be subject to increased licensing fees and government regulation than other structures. Profits are taxed both at the corporate level and again when distributed to shareholders.

Business Structures

C Corporation Continued-Shareholders are not personally liable for corporate obligations unless corporate formalities have not been observed; such formalities provide evidence that the corporation is a separate legal entity from its shareholders. Failure to do so may open the shareholders to liability of the corporation's debts. Corporate formalities include:

- issuing stock certificates
- holding annual meetings
- recording the minutes of the meetings
- electing directors or ratifying the status of existing directors Corporations should always be assisted by a qualified attorney."

(www.sba.gov)

Sub Chapter S Corporation (Inc. or Ltd.)

"This structure is identical to the C Corporation in many ways, but offers avoidance of double taxation. If a corporation qualifies for S status with the IRS, it is taxed like a partnership; the corporation is not taxed, but the income flows through to shareholders who report the income on their individual returns."

(www.sba.gov)

Preferred Business Structure   Rationale
Pros of Selected Business Structure   Cons of Selected
Business Structure   Resources

*Note-You can change from one business structure to another structure as long as you follow the guidelines set by your state.

Incorporation Steps

- You will need to come up with a business name. Keep it simple and general, especially if you choose to work in different settings and with different populations. For example, you do not want to use a name like, "Gero-Therapy" if you will possibly work in settings with middle-aged adults or in pediatric settings. My business name is Therapeutic Solutions of NC and it is universal for any therapy setting. However, a few people have told me that they thought I sold massage potions, which is not the case! Think about how your business name will sound to the general public. Will they know what service you are providing based on the name? Also, think about how your business name will be utilized, as a web address and email?

- You will then need to register your business name.

This step is required so that multiple businesses are not operating under the same name. For example, another company was using the name, "Therapeutic Solutions" in my state so my business name had to be modified and is actually Therapeutic Solutions of NC. The Secretary of State recommends several strategies to search the availability of a business name. You can also check the names of corporations by doing a corporations "search" on the Secretary of State home page. To find your secretary of state, you can do a simple internet search for : Your State Name (NC for me)Secretary of State. You can also do this same search onwww.irs.gov. Procedures and costs will vary from state to state and county to county.

- Once you have chosen your business name, choose a type of corporation. It is recommended that you check your state's Corporations Act to ensure that you are compliance with the state's regulations. (See Appendix C- NC GS 55). Next, you will go to your state's secretary of state and fill out the appropriate incorporation paperwork and pay the corresponding fees. Despite how easy the paper work now seems to me, I know that some people would prefer that a professional handle all of this start-up paperwork. There are plenty of companies and attorneys that will do this for you as long as you are willing to pay the money.

- You will need to file for an employment identification number (EIN) for your business through the IRS. The EIN is like a social security number for your business. You will fill out and submit an SS4 form and the IRS will issue you a number. You can now complete this form online: https://www.irs.gov/businesses/small-businesses-self-employed/apply-for-an-employer-identification-number-ein-online

Web address for instructions on filling out SS4 form: http://www.irs.gov/pub/irs-pdf/iss4.pdf(See Appendix D)

Web address for the paper SS4 form: http://www.irs.gov/pub/irs-pdf/fss4.pdf

- Are you done yet? No, You will need to file an annual report each year. The department of the secretary of state can again give you the information regarding keeping your corporation current. You will receive a notice regarding the need to fill out your annual report. However, if you do not receive it, you are still responsible for completing the report annually. In NC, I fill out a simple one-page report annually (cleverly called the Annual Report) online and pay around $200 to maintain my LLC status.

Ten Simple Steps to Independent Contracting

- You will still fill out a W-9 for each agency in which you contract for tax purposes. You fill this form out instead of the usual employee tax forms. (See Appendix F) for a sample copy of a W-9. Again you can learn more about the W-9 form onwww.irs.gov. See Appendix D

Web address for instructions on filling out aW-9 form-

http://www.irs.gov/pub/irs-pdf/iw9.pdf

Web address for W-9 form- http://www.irs.gov/pub/irs-pdf/fw9.pdf

- You will use your employment identification number instead of your social security number on the W-9 form

- You will still receive a 1099 instead of a W-2 at the end of year, which will state the total amount of money you made for the year. The 1099 will have your business name and your EIN on it.

Step 4-Get Insured!

You will need to obtain professional liability insurance since you will not have coverage from your contracting agency.

"Professional Liability Insurance protects you against covered claims arising from real or alleged errors or omissions, including negligence, in the course of your professional duties. Remember, legal defense and settlement costs are paid in addition to your limits of liability."

www.personal-plans.com/aota

Your contract agreements will state the amount of coverage that you will need per year and per incident. Every contract that I have had and have now requires professional liability insurance. Do not panic regarding paying for this coverage because it is very inexpensive. I currently use Healthcare Providers Service Organization (HSBO) and I pay only $211 per year for $1,000,000 of coverage per incident and 3,000,000 aggregate. MARSH Affinity has a comparable rate.

Fortunately, I have never had to use my liability insurance and I have been told by insurance agencies that occupational therapists rarely get sued. Nevertheless, no matter what your vocation is, you always want to have adequate coverage in the event that it is ever needed.

You can easily do an internet search for a list of companies that provide professional liability insurance to allied health professionals. Examples of companies with Professional Liability Insurance are listed below.

HSBO- http://www.hpso.com/

MARSH AFFINITY- http://www.seaburychicago.com/

We also now have general liability insurance which is a couple of thousand dollars per year. General liability insurance was required when we moved into our new office space. As its name states, it covers general liabilities, such as someone slipping in your office and not professional liabilities resulting from clinical service provision. The aforementioned insurances also have general liability policies. I personally however use a local agent for this policy.

You may also need to obtain worker's compensation insurance. I do not have worker's compensation but have used it in the past as it was required by an agency in which I was contracting with. Since, I no longer have this contract and do not have four or more employees, I have dropped the policy.

When I had the policy, the cost was based on my expected payroll and we even received a refund because we over-projected. I was told that we would owe if we had under-projected. The quotes I received for worker's compensation insurance were from $1500 to $2500 per year. We ended up paying the latter! You will need to check your state law regarding worker's compensation insurance and the contract agency's expectancy regarding this coverage. I recommend getting several quotes for this insurance if you decide to obtain it. Also, check with your professional organizations to find out if any of them have partnerships with companies that provide worker's compensation insurance.

You may be wondering what happens if you are injured on a job and do not have worker's compensation insurance. You might think that this issue would be a concern for the contracting agency. Yes, it is a concern and for this reason, the contracting agencies that I have worked with specify that they are not liable for any work-related injuries. It also states that I must understand that I will have to pay all costs for any injuries that occur on the job. I am responsible for signing this contract and I have to take full responsibility for work-related injuries. Thus, you may choose to obtain worker's compensation insurance even if it is not required for the sole purpose of having insurance coverage in the event that you are injured while working or disability insurance.

Finally, you may want to obtain other types of insurance coverage for yourself and family if you are single or do not have coverage under your spouse's or partners employer. These are insurances that an employer typically offers at discounted prices or free to their employees. Of course, all of these insurances are optional. A list of insurances that you may want to consider are listed below:

- Health insurance
- Dental insurance
- Vision insurance
- Life insurance

- Disability insurance
- Accident/Injury
- Long-term care insurance

The marketplace: https://www.healthcare.gov/get-coverage/

Therapeutic Solutions has a list of affiliate agencies that we have partnered with to help you meet all of your insurance needs.

Please contact us for more info!

Step 5: An Accountant and Attorney are Your Friends-Develop a Rapport

Because you will be responsible for paying your own taxes, you may want to consider getting an accountant to set-up a simple program for your business finances. You are required to pay your estimated taxes quarterly (four times per year: April, June, September and Jan. of the following year). If you are small and contracting as an individual, it is unlikely that you will need an accountant every month but that will be your discretion. The more organized you are the better off you will be in terms of financial management, including providing information in the event that you are audited.

Your Team-Accountant and Attorney

It is pertinent that you keep track of your income and expenses. You have several options for keeping track of your business finances. You can be very professional using a computer program, such as Quick Books or you can keep it very simple, such as using a basic one-subject notebook or an excel program. I used a one-subject notebook for two years. I had a page for each month of the year. I then put my income in one column and my expenses in another column for each month of the year.

Next, I recorded my net monthly income at the bottom of each page. I placed twenty-four long envelopes in the notebook. I designated two envelopes for each month. The envelopes were labeled "income" and "expenses." I put corresponding check stubs in the "income" envelope and corresponding business expense receipts in the "expenses" notebook. My income and expenses information in the envelopes matched the income and expense information recorded in the tablets. A business checking account connected to Quick books does these steps for you. It can also log your mileage using a cell phone app.

Do I need to open up a business checking account?

A business checking account is not required. However, I do recommend having a separate account for your contracting income, weather it is just a regular personal checking account or an actual business account. It is good business skills to keep your personal income from your contracting income so that you can have accurate records of your contracting profits. If you are incorporated, you can contact your bank's business center and give them your EIN (as well as other information) to create a formal "business account." The internal revenue service will have access to your business account records so again I emphasize maintaining good records. You can also obtain a business credit card to start building business credit. An advantage of a business credit card is that these cards typically have low interest rates

Your Team-Accountant and Attorney

It is a good idea to have a rapport with an attorney to look over contracts, provide legal advice as needed, and represent you in the event that you ever have to go to court. Attorneys can also explain your legal obligations as a health care business entity. In my experience, I have never had to use an attorney besides having one look over an amended contract and asking some basic legal questions. The utilization of legal services is at your discretion. However, if you will be directly billing insurance, such as Medicare and Medicaid, you will need to have someone available that has a good understanding of the insurance companies policies, procedures, regulations and legal penalties.

I used to use a prepaid legal service but now use a local attorney. When we were smaller, I paid a monthly standard payment in exchange for free and discounted legal services. Currently, I pay per service for a reputable attorney which is more expensive but helps me sleep at night. Professional OT organizations may also have recommendations for attorneys and again, you can easily do an internet search for attorneys in your area that work with health care professionals. A key word to use when doing your search is "Health Law."

http://www.legalshield.com

Step 6-Determine Your Rate-What's the Plan?

Many therapists have told me that they are unsure about the rate that they should charge if they decide to become an independent contractor. I have been asked several times, "What is the going rate?" Well rates vary based on many factors. Some contractors charge per hour, some charge per assessment and others charge per day.

You and the contract agency will have to come an agreement regarding a billable rate that is satisfactory and economical to both of you. Remember that a contractual rate is much higher than an employee rate because employees receive benefits and a portion of their taxes are paid by the employer. A contractor must take these additional expenses into consideration when determining their billable rate.

Show Me the Money-A Negotiable Rate

This is a hypothetical scenario and is not meant to be fully comprehensive in nature. Each individual will need to determine their income needs and thoroughly understand the associated business expenses.

- How much money do you want to make after taxes and expenses?

I am interested in making $1000 per week after taxes and expenses. This amount is $52,000 per year.

- What expenses will I include in my rate?
  - Health insurance-$250 per month= $3000 per year
  - Dental insurance-$60 per month=$720 per year
  - Accident insurance-$20 per month=$240 per year
  - Professional Liability insurance=$300 per year
  - Accountant annual fee-$300 per year
  - Attorney annual fee-$350year
  - Annual report to maintain corporation status-$200

Total Expenses to be included in contract rate=$5110; Always round up =$5500

You may want to also consider vacation and sick days, as well as travel expenses and other business expenses. Because I typically only work two days per week, I do not add vacation and sick days in my rate. I simply work more days the week before or after my vacation or sick time. I also do not include travel expenses because with only two days of travel, this expense is minimal. I will however write off my travel expense, it is just not included in my rate. Also consider office supplies and adaptive equipment expenses unless you use the supplies at the facilities of the contract agency. You may want to include retirement and savings also.

The current total annual income I need is now $57,500. I will however pay taxes on the $52,000 (or less because of other tax write-offs). For the purpose of this example, we will say that I will be paying approximately 1/3 of my income in taxes. Therefore, I will need to make more than $52,000 to actually bring home $52,000 because a third is going to Uncle Sam. Look at the equation below to determine how much money I need to make in order bring home $52,000 after paying 1/3 in taxes.

X-1/3x=$52,000

Solve for x and x= $78,000

$78,000-(1/3 $78,000)=$52,000

$78,000-$26,000=$52,000

You will need $78,000 plus the $5500 in business expenses included in your rate for a total of: $83,500.

Now, how many hours would you like to work per week? I will say 30 hours per week. There are 52 weeks in a year so I will simply multiply 30 x 52 =1560 to get the total amount of hours that I would like to work per year. Then I divide the total desired income by the total yearly desired work hours.

$83,500/1560/hours = $53

$53 per hour at 30 hours per week will give you approximately $52,000 per year after you pay your expenses and taxes. Not bad, huh? You could also include three weeks of paid vacation by simply multiplying by 49 weeks per year instead of 52.

Now, it's your turn—Try it—Come up with your rates!

*Consider hiring a financial advisor to assist you with your financial planning as an independent contractor. I strongly recommend this expertise as I waited almost ten years before understanding the comprehensive financial needs that were required to be truly successful financially as a person and a business owner.

Step 7: Review or Write Your Contracts

As an IC, you and a representative from the contracting agency will sign a contract agreement. This agreement will include the terms and regulations that you must abide by while providing services to the contracting agency. The agency's responsibilities are also stated in this agreement. One must read this agreement carefully and I recommend having an attorney look over it for your protection. In most cases, agencies already have contract agreements in place. You may however what to modify the agreement based upon your needs and desires and recommendations from your attorney. In some cases, however agencies have never hired contractors and may ask you for a contract. I have had this experience two times and I did not re-invent the wheel. In other words, I reworded contract agreements that I had obtained from previous agencies. The length will depend on how detailed you and the agency would like to be. Again, I recommend hiring an attorney to look over your contracts. You may also want to consider having signatures notarized, particularly if you are working with a new or unfamiliar company. In my webinars and courses, I review some of the key things to consider in your contract agreements.

Step 8-Marketing

In terms of marketing, as an independent contractor I suggest doing as much as possible yourself. Remember that you are trying to earn money, not lose it. I know people who really get caught up on fancy business cards and brochures. These materials can be pretty expensive. As an independent contractor, I think you will be fine keeping it simple. However if you decide to expand beyond a solo independent contractor, then the investment for a marketer can be well worth the costs.

You can purchase software at a local office supply store and make your own business cards and brochures or use free online templates. I have purchased software for $9.99 that included templates for business cards, flyers, brochures and greeting cards. You can also purchase a package of business card or brochure paper for as cheap as $11.99. Many computers already have business templates available and you can also make customized business marketing materials at local office stores, such as Staples and online companies, such as Vista. Local department stores often have same day services for business cards and other products

The software programs are pretty simple. I actually have three different programs and I am technology challenged! However, I have not had a problem creating marketing materials using any of the step- by- step instructions. An advantage of creating your own marketing materials is that you can make cards and brochures with various styles for corresponding settings. If you are working with nursing facilities and home health agencies, you can personalize a card for each of these practice settings. You can also change your cards style at any time. Finally, you can print as needed. You may want to print out 20 cards now and 20 cards a year from now or you may want to print 50 now. It is totally up to you. If you purchase cards from a marketing company, you will likely have to purchase a minimum amount of cards, usually100+.

Websites are also a way in which you can market your independent contracting services. Websites however are much more expensive than business cards and brochures. You should ask yourself if you really need a website. As an independent contractor a simple online portfolio may suffice. There are many free and low cost website options online. Check out wix, weebly and homestead. A monthly fee may apply if you choose to create a personalized domain name. Hosting is the term used for keeping your site on the web. Therefore, you will need an agency to host your website. Shop around to get the lowest price! This same agency can probably also help you register your website's domain name (www.yourcompanyname.com).

Please contact tomeico@tsofnc.comif you are interested in obtaining further website design and consultation services through my business consultation and coaching services.

One of the cheapest and simplest ways to get your marketing materials to agencies is to simply mail your business cards and/or brochures (with website info. if applicable) to agencies that you would like to work. You can also give these materials out to vendors and therapists at continuing education workshops and professional events.

A press release with educational information can be a very inexpensive form of advertisement. You can even call the local news station and asked for an interview.

A final great way to market your services is to provide your services free of charge (particularly if it is a new service not provided by a traditional health care agency) or at a huge discount for a specified period of time. Once you have the opportunity to provide your services for people, those people will then tell people they know, and they will tell people they know.....and so on.

ELEVATOR PITCH-How will you pitch your business to a company in need of your services? Why should they choose you over the large staffing agencies?

Write it out: I am an independent contractor and I specialize in.... Benefits of using my contractual services include...

STEP 9-Consider Hiring Subcontractors if You Want to Expand

At some point, you may decide that you want to grow your company and hire more staff. You may decide that you want to work less and would rather divide the requested contract hours between yourself and another therapist. You can expand your company by hiring employees or hiring subcontractors. Because I have had as many as five subcontractors at once and found this route of growth fairly easy, I will outline the basic steps of hiring a subcontractor. I recommend starting out with 1-2 subcontractors and then adding more gradually. Below are some points that are relevant in regards to hiring subcontractors.

• Make sure that your contract states that it is OK to for you to hire subcontractors. Some contracts specifically state that subcontractors are not allowed.

• Create a contract agreement between your company and each subcontractor. This contract agreement should include the same terms of agreement that are stated in the contract between you/your company and the contract agency. I recommend having an attorney look over any contracts you/your company creates for subcontractors. The subcontractors should get a copy of the contract agreement that you signed with the contract agency (minus the contracted rate)

• Subcontractors should be responsible for their taxes and insurances because they are not your employees.

• You/your company will handle all administration communication with the contract agency. The subcontractor will communicate with you directly regarding billing and other administrative issues. The subcontractor will also turn billing invoices into you/your company directly and you/your company will turn this paperwork into the contract agency.

• You will get paid from the contract agency and then you will be responsible for paying the subcontractor/s.

• Ensure that you have enough income to pay the subcontractor even if you do not get paid by the contract agency. Been there, done that. Agencies have held checks before and it was not pretty when I was not prepared. Consider having a 3 to 6 month payment emergency fund.

• Subcontractors are typically responsible for continuing education. You can provide continuing education but it should be at cost. Remember that the subcontractor is a separate entity from you/your company.

• Ensure your contract rate covers enough money for you to pay the subcontractor and make enough profit to pay yourself for the additional responsibility of having subcontractors. You don't want to request a rate of $50 per hour and pay your subcontractor $50 per hour because you will not make any money for time used to answer subcontractor questions, follow-up on subcontractor work, proof subcontractor invoices, market, time to secure contracts, etc.

- Understand that you are ultimately responsible for the contract that has been created between you/your company and the contract agency. Therefore you need to be aware of the subcontractor's performance. You may not necessarily have to supervise the subcontractor/s directly but will need to be informed and aware of their performance.

- You will need to keep a file on each of your subcontractors with required documents per your contract agreement.

- Consider a buy-out clause in the contract in the event that the contractor wants to become an employee for the agency.

Step 10-Go Get Some Contacts!!!

OK, occupational therapists, are you ready? Now that you have these basic steps to independent contracting, get busy! You CAN still work if you need flexibility as a mom, a dad, a student or just someone who wants the freedom that comes with independent contracting and you CAN bring home a nice income! I believe I mentioned in the beginning of this booklet that I am ALWAYS thinking of new businesses for therapists. Below are a list of some sample contract ideas.

- *Low vision in long term care settings*
- *Low vision in hospitals*
- *Outpatient low vision*
- *Low vision with home health agencies*
- *Low vision with optometrists or retina specialists*
- *Hand therapy at family practices (I previously worked at a family practice that reserved a day for a podiatrist. It was very successful. I believe a hand therapist at a family practice would be even more successful)*
- *Developmental Disability Group Home Consultation*

- *Universal Design Consultant for Architects*
- *Home Modification Consultant Senior Housing Communities*
- *Ergonomic Consultant in a variety of settings*
- *Mental Health Services at Clubhouses*
- *Mental Health at Day Programs*
- *Alzheimer's Specialist at Adult Day Programs*
- *Feeding and Swallowing Specialists in NICUs and in early intervention*
- *Fall Prevention Specialist in long term care settings*
- *Fall Prevention Specialist in home health*
- *Tele therapy*
- *Functional mobility*
- *Concussion prevention*
- *Yoga and physical therapy studio*
- *Military Contractual services*
- *Wheelchair and Seating specialist in rehab. and long-term care settings*
- *Driving Specialists in outpatient settings*
- *Driving Specialists in long term care settings*
- *Community-based driving specialist*
- *Lifestyle Redesign Specialist in senior apartments for the elderly*
- *Assistive Technology Specialist*
- *Vocational Assessment Specialist*
- *Splinting and Orthotic Specialist*
- *Program Planner in Community Based Settings*
- *Visual-Perceptual Specialist for Learning Centers*
- *Sensory Integration Specialist for a variety of settings*
- *Adaptive Cranial Helmet Specialist*
- *Augmentative Communication Specialist at group homes*

- School system, daycare and early intervention contractor
- Bi-lingual therapists-big need!!
- Besides specialties, one can propose contracting at virtually any agency that needs your skills...

At a contractual rate of $90 per hour 40 hours per week, at 50 weeks a year, gross income can be around $160,000.

If you add full time subcontractors at 50% profit (so $80,000 annually based on the above scenario), gross income can equal around one million dollars with 10 contractors.

Please note that I am emphasizing profits here because I am an advocate of increasing revenues for the purpose of increasing service. If you put service first, the money will follow. Much of my company's profit has been turned over as an investment for adding services for underserved populations because there are so many needs! You can help meet those needs also!

Good luck and please let me know if this booklet has been helpful to you and if you would recommend any changes. Email me at tomeico@tsofnc.com

If you would like additional consultation or coaching, I am happy to help YOU! I am dedicated to educating and advocating for health and human service entrepreneurs! In addition to consulting and coaching, I am also now hosting webinars and teaching courses to help you create your dream business that affords you a wonderful lifestyle while making a profit and serving others. These webinars and courses have bonus content including information on federal government contracting, tips for negotiating a contract, key contractual terms, group contracts, mastering networking and MORE! www.faisonconsulting.com for more information about upcoming events!

Subscribe to our newsletter for monthly information and inspiration:

https://faisonconsulting.us3.listmanage.com/subscribe?u=cd524a3bb563a95d8b4e91619&id=860463a4bf

Final Thoughts:

I am an occupational being and so are you. You deserve to work in a way that is fulfilling to you and your family. You deserve to love your work and your life!

I am a wife, a mom, a daughter, a sister, a ministry participant, an advocate, a runner, a writer, an educator, a real estate investor and a business consultant and certified business coach dedicated to helping you create your dream businesses! It CAN be done because I AM LIVING PROOF!

Go Get Some Contracts!

www.faisonconsulting.com

Create opportunities, tell your mind what to think and believe that you CAN!

Blessings, Tomeico Faison

www.ingramcontent.com/pod-product-compliance
Lightning Source LLC
Chambersburg PA
CBHW030536220526
45463CB00007B/2857